30 Days to a

Better You

Tiffaney Beverly-Malott

Insight Publishing
Sevierville, TN

Insight Publishing
647 Wall Street
Sevierville, Tennessee 37738

Dedication

This book is dedicated to the hundreds of women that participated in my first annual Women's Event in Chicago, Illinois. The desire in each of you to be your very best pulled the very best out of me. Thank you. I look forward to us all growing together.

Acknowledgements

I thank God, for equipping and allowing me to do what I love to do. A sincere, heartfelt thank you goes to my husband, John, for keeping me focused and believing in me every step of the way. To all the people in my life that have been my mentors, teachers and friends, I appreciate you so much. There are too many of you to name; but for your kindness, I am forever indebted to you all.

Table of Contents

Purpose

This book is a result of me listening to a soft voice that spoke to my spirit. I was preparing for the first Women's Event I had ever organized. It was a huge undertaking. We flew 12 incredible women into Chicago from all around the country. They represented a very rare segment of our society today: women that earn a 6-figure income from home. Each woman was asked to train on a specific topic and to give assignments to the 500+ women attending the event to take home. That way they could apply the great lessons they received to their lives. God told me that my assignment was to be a 30-day devotional book.

I know how easy it is to receive life-changing information and do nothing with it. You need someone to help you apply those lessons to your life. You need an unwavering voice, a committed friend, a tireless workout partner to be there to push you to achieve your goals. I have been blessed with these types of people all my life. I want to be that person for you.

I heard a well-known pastor tell the Old Testament Bible story of Esther. He described Esther's dismal situation. I had heard that part of the story before. But he went into detail about Esther's relative, Mordecai, who took care of her when her parents died. He believed in Esther when no one else did, including Esther. Even though she was a poor orphan, he spoke words of motivation, inspiration and success into her seemingly hopeless circumstances. Eventually, those words took shape in Esther's heart, her mind and her life. She became the Queen of her land and saved her people from death.

I feel many of us are like Esther. Our situation seems dire. Our future looks bleak. But all we need is a Mordecai! We need someone who sees more in us than we see in ourselves. We crave that special person who tells us our past does not have to dictate our future. We are looking for someone who wants to pour into us for the sole purpose of helping us become better. That is the purpose of this book. I would like to be that person for you. I am now asking for your permission. Will you allow me to be your Mordecai? If the answer is 'yes', let's begin our journey together.

Introduction

You may be asking yourself, "Who is Tiffaney Beverly-Malott? Who said she was qualified to help anyone become better?" I would like to answer those questions. I was born a poor, black child in Winston-Salem, North Carolina... Just kidding. I won't take you back that far.

Who is Tiffaney Beverly-Malott? I'm an ex-jelly maker. You read it right. I made jelly for a living. I worked in a factory on third shift in Memphis, Tennessee. I was employed as a supervisor in food manufacturing for five years. I graduated from Mississippi Valley State University with a business degree. I had a job, an apartment, a Volkswagen Jetta and student loans. I was just like a lot of other people. There was nothing extraordinary about me; except what happened to me in the year 2000. I was introduced to a home-based business opportunity that changed my life, Pre-Paid Legal Services.

I know, I know. Those things don't work. This is another one of those books. But wait, before you close your mind and this book, let me ask you a question. If I told you that because of Pre-Paid Legal, I am a 35-year old woman that earns a multiple six-figure income from home, would you read more? Yes? Then keep reading. I got involved with Pre-Paid Legal just to make some extra money without getting a second job. It turned into much more than that. I walked away from my job after only working PrePaid Legal for five months. I was earning a six-figure income three years later. I am now married to John Malott, another PPL associate, and together we work from home and earn a multiple-six figure income. We are millionaires at the ages of 35 and 37; and I was once a jelly-maker and he was a janitor.

This book is not about Pre-Paid Legal. But if it weren't for Pre-Paid Legal, I would not be writing this book. What does my journey with this company have to do with becoming a better you? That's the first tip. You have to do something different to get something different. You can't get better if you aren't willing to change your situation for the better. Even when people don't understand, change anyway. That's what I did; and I now have new philosophies, new friends, and a new lifestyle. I have true joy in my life for the very first time. I am doing all the things I love to do. None of these things would have happened if I was still making jelly.

I can help you be a better you because I've done it myself. I made one decision, stuck with it and my life shifted 180 degrees. I was living a life of mediocrity. Today I live a life of victory. Deciding to become better doesn't mean you're bad; it just means you know there is more in you and you want to share it. It means you want to live your best life and help those you love do the same.

There you have it. That's my story. Do I know what I'm talking about? Can I help you become a better you? Well, you'll never know if you don't decide to take the journey with me. So, turn the page…

Getting Started

You already know the areas you want to improve in your life. I'm not here to tell you what to do; I'm just here to urge you to do it. This book is going to be a daily push for you; but it is also a journal for you to record your progress toward your goals over the next thirty days.

Paul J. Meyer, one of my mentors, teaches that we must have balance in all areas of our lives. If you lack discipline in one area of your life, then eventually that area will affect the other areas of your life. Mr. Meyer separated our lives in six areas. I'd like to share with you what he shared with me.

1. Physical & Health-your overall physical health; exercise, eating habits, etc.
2. Social & Cultural-your contributions to your community
3. Spiritual & Ethical-your faith and core values
4. Family & Home-your relationship with your spouse or significant other and children
5. Financial & Career-your money situation and your vocation
6. Mental & Educational-your philosophies and personal growth

We can't neglect any one of these areas. If we do, that area will eventually adversely affect other areas.

I would like you to write down ONE goal for each of the six areas that you would like to achieve over the next thirty days. It doesn't have to be earth shattering. It just needs to be a small step in the right direction. Maybe you don't exercise every day and you know you need to. Set a goal to walk fifteen minutes per day. Maybe you need to spend less time at work and more time with your family. Put in your schedule thirty minutes of family time every day. Maybe you don't pay yourself first; make a goal to pay yourself before you pay anyone else at each pay period. You get the picture. Working on one small thing in each area for thirty days will lead to more positive changes in your life. Eventually, these small changes will lead to a better you living a better life.

It's time for you to write your thirty-day goals. What small changes would you like to make in each area of your life? Write them down. Let me say that again. Write them down! Sometimes we try to keep our goals in our heads. That is the biggest mistake we can make. The Bible says, "Write the vision, make it plain." Habakkuk 2:2-3. Your goals must me personal, possible and profitable. Let me break that down. Your goals must be for you, you must be able to achieve them, and they must make you better in some way when you achieve them.

Before you write your goals, I've written my goals to give you an example:

1. Physical & Health: I eat six small meals per day.
2. Social & Cultural: I read to school children for one hour every week.
3. Spiritual & Ethical: I read my Bible every day and spend quality time with God.
4. Family & Home: I tell my husband and children how awesome they are every day.
5. Financial & Career: I helped ten people get their first check this month in PPL.
6. Mental & Educational: I read one hour per day.

If you look at my goals, you see they are written in past or present tense. I wrote those goals as if they have happened already or they happen every day. Why did I write my goals that way? My subconscious believes whatever I tell it. So, I'm telling my subconscious that I already eat six small meals per day, when I only eat three times per day right now. Is that a little tricky? Maybe it is. But because I am the master programmer of my future, I will give my subconscious the language it needs to help me succeed. You must do the same. You must also give yourself a deadline. I've already provided the deadline. We only have thirty days. So let's get going! Write your goals here:

Physical & Health   _____

_____

Social & Cultural   _____

_____

Spiritual & Ethical   _____

_____

Family & Home _____

_____

Financial & Career _____

_____

Mental & Educational _____

_____

    I put in some extra lines, because I know some of you write big. Now that your goals are written, I suggest you write them again. This time, write your goals bigger; (we have provided blank sheets in the back of this book), and put them somewhere you have to see them every day, like the refrigerator or your bathroom mirror. This will serve as a constant reminder for you to stick to your goals. But it will also serve as a reminder for your subconscious mind as well. Your subconscious mind believes everything you tell it, good or bad. So if you tell yourself that you are going to spend more time with your family; your subconscious mind believes it and works on you from the inside out to make that happen. If you don't tell your subconscious mind that you're going to pay yourself first, you'll keep doing the same thing you've been doing. We must program our subconscious mind with good things. If we don't, the negative influences of the world will program it for us.

    Now that we have written our goals, it's time to get started. Consciously decide right now that you will achieve your goals. The next step is to read Day One. Becoming better is just that simple; making a decision, taking the first steps to make it happen and sticking with it.

    After you read each day, write down how you're doing and how you're feeling. Chronicle your activities, your successes and your failures. Everything you write down is important. It is all part of your journey to becoming a better you. The joy is in the journey, not the destination. So enjoy it, relish it and grow from it.

Day One
Keep God First

"But seek first the kingdom of God and His righteousness, and all things shall be added to you."

Matthew 6:33

I realize there are many different faiths represented by those reading this. You may have a different name for Your Creator. But, I'm sure we all agree, there is a Higher Power. Since I'm writing this, I'm going to call Him GOD. As a woman, I love a strong, take charge man! So, God it is!

The scripture says to seek Him first and ALL things shall be added to you. So, to keep it simple, if we put Him first, we'll get everything else. Let's go over how to seek Him first.

With all the things we have to balance in our lives, it's very easy to say we don't have time. The first thing we must do is make time for God. I'm not trying to diminish God's role in our lives by saying put Him on your schedule. I am saying you schedule everything else: your job/business, your children, your spouse, your physical fitness. You need to put God on your schedule. He's the reason you have a schedule anyway. Having a set time will create discipline and a habit. Soon, you will look forward to your time with Him.

Study His word. My mother used to tell me the scripture, "study to show thyself approved." Being a sweet person and a loyal spouse is just not enough. You must know His word. That way, God's instructions can always be in you, no matter what you're going through during your day.

Live His word. Work to take what you've learned and apply it to your life. Take a scripture and work to be the living embodiment of that word. Nobody's perfect. I've learned striving to be better brings me closer to God.

Teach it to your children. Make God's word a regular topic of conversation in your home. That way, God can be at the center of your family life. Your children will take the goodness and guidance of His word with them every day.

I'm not an expert. I'm just someone on the journey. I know from personal experience that for ultimate success, this is the first step. You have to have Him at the head of your life to have a great life. A good spiritual walk is part of a balanced life. Lack of discipline in this area of your life, will soon affect all other areas of your life.

Day Two
First Things First

"In case of a decrease in cabin pressure an oxygen mask will come down. Please place the mask over your nose and mouth. Put your mask on first before you put the mask on someone else."

Safety briefing done by flight attendants

In the book *You...*, the author, Frances Wilshire teaches The Law of Spiritual Equilibrium, which means half to yourself and half to the world. She teaches, "You must first give your entire attention to the improvement, the knowledge and the development of yourself. You must spend your time, your effort, and your money first on yourself. For you must first have the strength, vitality, wisdom or money to be able to give and thereby fulfill the second half of the law." She said, "You cannot take out of a bag what is not in it. You cannot give unless you have something to give."

"Everywhere we see the mother who gives all to her children. On the surface it seems to be very noble and unselfish. But let's follow it through and see the results. The mother loses her health, her looks, maybe her money. In the end, she even loses the respect and admiration of the very children for who she has given all. People say, 'What selfish and unappreciative children.' The mother is to blame. She violated the fundamental law of her own nature, The Law of Equilibrium."

When I first read this, I was in shock. I thought, "There is nothing wrong with sacrificing yourself for those you love. " But I get it now. Frances Wilshire is

3

right. Are we really helping anyone by neglecting ourselves? In a world where people need positive role models, why wouldn't we take care of ourselves so our children can look up to us; instead of some bulimic, anorexic, pill-popping, drunk driving, no talent having super model turned TV personality?

First things must come first...you. Today we put ourselves first. This is not being selfish. You can't care for your spouse, your children, your family or your friends if you aren't the best you can be. For the next 29 days, starting today, you will take care of you. That way you can take better care of the others you love.

We can't help, influence, empower, inspire or equip someone else if we aren't a living example. Today we start the process to becoming that example. You must put you on your TO DO list. Treat yourself to lunch, a movie, a massage, a bubble bath, quiet time, a nap or a good book. It doesn't have to be expensive or extravagant. It just has to be for you.

Set YOU goals; goals that will make you happier and better. Others may not understand or appreciate them; but it doesn't matter. They are your goals, not theirs. In your hectic life, remember to set time aside for you to be physically fit, spiritually lifted and professionally charged. Remember, as much as you love your family, you aren't helping them if you aren't helping yourself.

_____

_____

_____

_____

_____

_____

_____

Day Three
Start Now!

"You don't have to be great to start…you just have to start to be great."

To begin. To quickly come to life. To spring forth. All of these are definitions of the word start. My definition of start: you, today, right now, taking the first steps to being all you were put here to be.

Why shouldn't you start now? You don't have time? That's a reason you need to start. You have children? That's another reason you need to start. You don't know what you're doing? That's just another reason to get started. Let me give you some more reasons: your spouse, your finances, and your demanding job. All of these are reasons to get started now!

We can't achieve any of our goals if we don't start. Don't worry about how bad your first presentation will be; or how tired you'll be when you walk or run that first mile; or how bad your finances will look when you take the first steps to get them in order. Don't focus on any of that! Remember, the journey of a thousand miles begins with a single step. Focus on the journey and how your first step will be only one of a thousand successful steps.

Don't berate yourself for wobbly first steps. Don't give up because you take your first steps and fall. You didn't do that to your children. Now they run all over the place, you can't keep up with them! Because of your love and encouragement, they didn't give up when they tried and failed. The fell, got up, and tried again. They were able to see those first attempts at walking for what they were, the beginning. They didn't focus on the start, they got laser focused on the finish.

I'm asking you not to focus on your start; focus on your finish. Imagine yourself at the finish line. Just remember, you've got to get out of the starting blocks to get there.

Day Four
Keep Your Goals in Front of You!

"Failures do what is tension relieving, while winners do what is goal achieving."
Dennis Waitley

Write down your goals in the present tense and make them specific. Put them everywhere. On your refrigerator, on your mirror, on your screensaver, everywhere!

Remember, your goals must be: possible, personal and profitable.

This will help you develop a burning desire. Constantly reminding yourself of your goals will keep you committed. But also, seeing them in the present tense, as if they have already taken place, convinces your subconscious that it's already done. So you start to act and think in a more successful way. It's kind of tricking your subconscious. Your subconscious believes whatever it's told, positive or negative. Then it goes to work on making that a reality.

So if you tell yourself you earn a multiple six-figure from home; you drive a black, Mercedes Benz CLS 55 AMG; you married your best friend in your dream wedding in Key West, (oops, sorry, that's my life); then your subconscious will cause you to become what it takes to make that happen. And it will happen. It did for me. It will for you.

Day Five
Surround Yourself with Positive People

"It is vitally important that the choices we make are positively positive in nature."

One of the best things about life is that we get to choose what we do and with whom we associate. We must choose to be around optimistic, upbeat people. We have to get away from the naysayers and dream stealers. You know who they are. Everything they say is negative. They can't see the good in anything.

But then there is another group. The 'yes, but' people. They agree with you, so they seem positive; but they always point out the negative. In their minds, they aren't pessimistic, they're realistic. It reminds of me a story I heard...

There were two farmers. One was positive, one was negative. One day, the two farmers went goose hunting together and the positive farmer brought along his new bird dog. He was so proud of that dog; he couldn't wait to show him off. The positive farmer, the negative farmer and the bird dog went out in a small boat and waited. Before long, a big goose flew overhead. BOOM! The positive farmer brought the bird down in the middle of the lake. He turned to his negative farmer friend and said, "Now watch what this dog can do." The dog jumped out of the boat and ran <u>on top of the water</u>, picked up the goose, ran back all the way <u>on top of the water</u>, and put the bird down perfectly in the boat.

9

The positive farmer was grinning from ear to ear. He turned to his negative friend and said, "What did you think of that?" The negative farmer shook his head in disgust. "Just what I thought," he said. "That dog can't even swim!"

Of course that story is just a joke; but you know those types of people all too well. They affect your mindset and ultimately your success. You must learn to disassociate. That means get away from them. Cut them off. That's right. Have nothing to do with them. Deciding to get away from these negative individuals and surround yourself with positive people will further your chances of success.

I know some of these people may be close to you. They are your friends and family members. You can't just cut them off. Then you must limit your associations with them. Spend less time with these individuals. Just become too busy or engaged in other activities. You can't let them put a damper on your spirits. Get around like minded people who only want to see you succeed.

For some of you, these naysayers and dream stealers live in the house with you. They are your spouse or significant other. So, disassociation is out of the question. Just plug into people that do believe in you and will speak positivity in your life. Try to get your spouse involved in your success journey. If that doesn't work, be strong enough to stay plugged in to those that do believe in you. So, one day your spouse can share in the rewards of your diligence.

Day Six
You Are What You Eat

"Tell me what you eat and I will tell you what you are."

Anthelme Brillat-Savarin

The above quote is the origin of the phrase: you are what you eat. Written in 1826, Brillat-Savarin was saying what we know is still true today: we are what we eat.

So what are you? A Frito? An Oreo cookie? A Big Mac? Or are you a Taco Supreme? Should we call you Diet Coke, Starbucks Latte double whip with chocolate sprinkles or Red Bull? Maybe you're something cute like Biscotti or Twix. Or should we call you Reese's for short?

We need a legal name change to Organic fruits and vegetables, baked not fried, and water not soda. I know it's not easy. Bad food is everywhere! We're bombarded with it! It's less expensive, it tastes good, and it's convenient. But that doesn't make it good for us. Obesity is on the increase globally and is set is to become the world's biggest health problem. Recent reports suggest that it may soon overtake cigarette smoking as a serious health risk.

Even if you're not overweight you still have to be careful what you eat. Type 2 Diabetes is at an all time high. Why? Sugar is in almost everything we eat! It's got another name too: high fructose corn syrup! Also, beware partially hydrogenated oils and white flour. This stuff will kill us and our children. I heard it said that the mother controls the health of the entire family. If she eats like crap, so will the kids. If you want a high quality of life for your ENTIRE family, change your eating habits today. Remember, if you play now, you'll pay later.

Some of you may be saying: 'what can I eat?' There are lots of healthy options. There are books, magazines, websites and TV shows that promote and teach how to live a healthier lifestyle. You can choose to listen or not.

Your body is like a priceless automobile that needs only the best fuel. Many of us give our cars better fuel than we give ourselves. We wouldn't dare put low octane gasoline in our high end car; but we put cheap fuel in our bodies at every meal.

Just remember, the most expensive thing is your own regret. It costs way more than a little discipline. I don't know about you, but I plan on being the friskiest, liveliest and sexiest septuagenarian around. (That's a person between 70 and 80 years old). I'm truly going to enjoy my golden years. The phrase is HEALTHY, wealthy and wise. I plan on being all three. You can too. Please don't think because you have lots of money, that everything else will fall in place. It won't. No amount of money is worth your health.

Make some wise health choices today, so you can live your best life tomorrow.

_____

_____

_____

_____

_____

_____

_____

_____

Day Seven
What Are You Willing to Give Up?

"The important thing is this…to be able to sacrifice what we are for what we would become."

Maharishi Mahesh Yogi

Are you willing to give up the you of today, to be the better you of tomorrow? Sacrificing who we are now means we have to shed some things. We have to shed some habits, associations, activities and thoughts. Are you willing to give up those things?

I don't know about you, but that's never been easy for me, even though I've been on this personal development journey for some years now. Giving up, to go up. I like the concept; it's just the giving up part that's been my struggle. I have to give up certain foods to be healthy, certain books and music to be wiser, and certain people to be better. That's a lot of giving up!

But I've learned to focus on the going up. I ask myself, 'Is the giving up worth how far up I'm going to go?' The answer was 'YES' every time.

Don't focus on the sacrifice, focus on the reward. Don't give everything up all at once. Give up one thing at a time. You'll see that you can live without it. You'll actually see how much better your life will be because of it.

The old Middle English meaning of the word sacrifice is "to make sacred". Many of us know sacrifice as 'to give up something'. That's correct, as well. But let's focus on the meaning, "to make sacred". Sacred means worthy of respect, veneration or worship. Our sacrifices today will make us worthy of the respect from others tomorrow.

That means we will be our children's role models; not the phony icons of pop culture. Our spouse will look at us as the ideal, not another person. Our counterparts in the workplace will look to us as the leaders, instead of someone else. All because we made the sacrifices today!

So when the sacrifices seem too hard to make, focus on the reward: being worthy of being respected and modeled by all of those around you!

Day Eight
How Bad Do You Want It?

"Are you eating, sleeping, dreaming with that one thing in mind?
Cause if you want it all,
You got to lay it all out on the line."
From "How Bad Do You Want it?" by Tim McGraw

You've set your goals. You have a plan to achieve them. How bad do you want it? Success ultimately begins with an idea; but desire turns ideas into reality. An idea can give you temporary inspiration; but burning desire helps you overcome the obstacles along the way.

I read, "When you're 100% committed to your goals, you move from hoping to knowing." Are you still hoping for success in all areas of your life? Or do you know that it can happen for you now?

Napoleon Hill, in his classic book, *Think and Grow Rich*, says a burning desire is one of the characteristics of the most successful. A burning desire is an urge, a passion, an inner drive that is so overwhelming that if denied will make you miserable no matter how much money or prestige you may have. The little known secret is that this desire is so all-encompassing that if embraced success is almost guaranteed. Do you have a burning desire? Do you an inner drive for your goals that is so overwhelming you will be miserable if you don't do anything else? And if you don't have that type of desire, can you get it? I believe the answer is, "Yes". This 30-day journey has steps that will help you get that burning desire you need to succeed.

15

The first thing you have to do is: Burn your Ships. This phrase comes from the Spanish Conquistador Hernando Cortez. He was committed to his mission of seizing the Aztec treasures in Mexico. His quest for riches is legendary. Because of Cortez's complete and total commitment, he convinced more than 500 soldiers and 100 sailors to set sail from Spain to Mexico to take the worlds' richest treasure. It was all or nothing! Failure was not an option for him, so he took that option away from his men. He ordered them to "Burn the ships!" In essence he told them," we win here or we die here." He gave them no escape. No fallback position. It was win or die. And win, they did. The men conquered the Aztecs and succeeded in something others had been unsuccessful in for six centuries.

Why did Cortez and his men succeed? They had no choice! Their backs were against the wall! Their level of commitment and motivation was high because they had no other option. What are the ships keeping you from achieving your goals? Whatever prevents you from achieving your goals are ships that need to be burned.

How bad do you really want it? Don't dismantle your ships or run them ashore. Burn your ships. And come out swingin'.

Day Nine
Don't Look Back

"You're not living to go backwards, you're living to go forward."

We've heard the saying, "your past doesn't have to equal your future." That's true. But sometimes we spend so much time looking back on our past, we can't see, much less, walk into our future.

Some of us live in the past because we think those were the best times of our lives. We have convinced ourselves that no other times will be better than 'the good old days'.

There are some of us that are living in our past of pain and suffering. We don't believe the future is bright because we keep reliving the dark yesterdays. Let those bad times go. It's over. You don't have to keep revisiting and reliving those bleak moments. You have too many good times ahead of you.

How do you stop living in the past? Appreciate where you are. You've got to be grateful for today, the present, the here and now! It doesn't matter if it's not all you want it to be. You have to be happy that you're here.

God didn't have to bless you with today. He could've left you in those good old days or those dark yesteryears. But He didn't. Show your appreciation by living every moment you have to the fullest. Start right now!

There are more days in your life. Some will be good, some not so good. But every one of your days is a gift that is special and irreplaceable. Stop looking back on days that are gone. Live today like the gift it is.

Tiffaney Beverly Malott

Day Ten
Use What You've Got

"Life is like a hand of cards. You have to play the hand you're dealt, you can't win by folding…"

Mike Conner

My mother used to tell me I had an ugly voice. She didn't mean any harm. I think I was using my voice at the wrong time and it was getting on her nerves. She told me my voice was too loud, too deep and too gravelly. So for years, I tried to speak in a higher octave.

I had a schoolmate tell me my smile was too big. She'd say, 'you don't need to show all of your teeth when you smile. It also makes your eyes crinkle up too much where you can't see them.' So I started smiling with just my lips, no teeth showing, and opening my eyes really wide. You know, like the Mona Lisa.

I had a teacher tell me, "If your parents aren't rich, you won't be either. You'll be just like them." So I became a supervisor in a manufacturing plant, just like my dad.

Then I read in *The Purpose Driven Life*, by Rick Warren, that I was planned for God's pleasure. That He deliberately chose every feature, prescribed every detail about me! And it all pleases Him! All I have to do is use it for His glory!

Now I speak around the country to audiences of thousands using my ugly voice. I use my crinkly-eyed, too big smile on every person I get a chance, to be a blessing to them and share God's goodness. And I use my parents' middle class life as a reason, not an excuse, to become wealthy and help others do the same.

What cards have you been dealt that you won't play because you think your hand's not good enough? Are you worried about everyone else's cards, instead of playing your own? Everything about you and everything that has happened to you is for a purpose.

Embrace it all and please God with what you do with it!

Day Eleven
GIVE

"Life's most urgent question is: What are you doing for others?"

Dr. Martin Luther King Jr.

Are you a giving person? Here's a test:

1. You've had a pack of tissues in your purse for a long time. Someone next to you is very upset and needs tissues. Do you give them:

    a.   the entire pack

    b.   one tissue, you may need some for later

2. When you buy gifts for others, which do you think of first?

    a.   the person

    b.   the price

3. Honestly, which would your friends and family members consider you:

    a.   a giver

    b.   a receiver

4. When you give or loan something to someone, do you talk about it all the time and remind everyone what you did?

    a.   no

    b.   yes

5. A friend has an emergency and really needs your help. It will require your time. Do you:

    a. tell them you'll be there, (you'll just rearrange your schedule later)

    b. tell them you've got to check your schedule first, you have too many things going on to just drop them

6. Who do you give to?

    a. family, friends, people with serious needs

    b. people who give to you

7. You have the opportunity to give a significant amount of money to help a lot of needy people. There are two stipulations: you can never tell anyone about it and you will never be repaid. Would you do it?

    a. yes, sign me up

    b. um, let me think about it

If you answered mostly A's, you're a giver. If you answered mostly B's…well, you're really cute and fun and all. You're just a little tight with what you've got and what you give.

2 Corinthians 9:7 says: "So let each one give as he purposes in his heart, not grudgingly or of necessity; for God loves a cheerful giver". That's not me saying it, that's THE WORD! No seriously, I'm not asking you to give to me or for me. I'm asking you to give for yourself.

Maya Angelou said," I have found that among its other benefits, giving liberates the soul of the giver." Elbert Hubbard said, "The love we give away is the only love we keep." Anne Frank said, "No one has ever become poor by giving."

If we pay attention, we keep seeing the wealthiest people in the world give obscene amounts of money away to help less fortunate people. But they stay wealthy! The more they give, the more they receive.

Maybe you don't have lots of money to give. That's okay. There are lots of things we can give besides money. We can give our time. Volunteer to help someone, a friend, a family member or an organization. Give some of those old clothes and toys away. Your trash can truly be someone else's treasure.

Give away some kindness. Just be nice to someone. Give that person you've overlooked a smile, a hug or a sincere thank you. You know who that person is. If it weren't for them your business, organization or home wouldn't be the same. There are many things we can give. Just look for opportunities to share your blessings with someone else. Remember: "A value of a man resides in what he gives and not in what he is capable of receiving." Albert Einstein.

_____

_____

_____

_____

_____

_____

_____

_____

_____

_____

Day Twelve
This Too Shall Pass

"You're not falling apart. Some things have just not come together yet."

Bishop Noel Jones

My father used to say, "This too shall pass." Even on his deathbed, he was telling me that the pain and suffering would soon be over. He reminded me difficult times don't last always. He was right, they don't. No matter what you're going through, embrace it, learn from it and know that it's just preparation for your next level.

See yourself on the other side of these difficult times. SMILE NOW for what's on the way. Get excited for the good times that are coming and for how much better equipped you will be from what you are experiencing now.

I had to drive through a terrible storm once. Golf ball sized hail was falling on the roof of my car. The wind was rocking my little Volkswagen Jetta. I couldn't see three feet in front of me. My friend riding with me told me to pull over until the storm passed. Other cars were pulling over on the side of the road waiting for the storm to end. But I kept going. I had to slow down, a lot. I went from 60 mph, to 50 to 35 to 20mph. At one point, I was going 10 mph! I could've walked faster! But I refused to stop. I kept moving forward, passing cars that had pulled over on the side of the road. We crept on for awhile following the lines on the road. Little by little, we plugged on. Eventually, I was able to drive a little faster, then a little faster. Before I knew it, I was back up to 55 mph. All of sudden, the storm was gone and the sun was shining brightly. Right in front of me was the most beautiful rainbow I had ever seen. I was so happy to have made it through the storm.

I thought about all the other drivers still in the storm. They stopped moving forward, they pulled over to side of the road and gave up. They opted to wait for the storm to pass, instead of pushing through the storm. So they had to endure the hail, the wind and the rain even longer because they chose to give up and give in, instead of pressing forward.

Difficult times will pass, eventually. But they go by faster if you PUSH through to the sunshine on the other side.

_____

_____

_____

_____

_____

_____

_____

_____

_____

_____

_____

_____

_____

_____

_____

_____

_____

Day Thirteen
Keep Your Eyes on the Prize

"Make your challenges temporary, but your vision permanent."

As you stick to this 30-day plan, challenges will come your way. There will be obstacles. It will seem like all hell has broken loose. And it has...because hell doesn't want you getting any better. Just remember that these challenges are temporary and necessary. Leonardo DaVinci said, "Obstacles cannot crush me; every obstacle yields to stern resolve." He refused to let obstacles get the best of him. He knew that challenges always concede to firm purpose and determination.

You must make your vision permanent. No matter how bad your situations may seem, just see your life as it will be. It will come to pass.

Your overcoming these challenges and obstacles is just proof of your desire, determination and your destiny. Keep your eye on the prize! Keep your goals in front of you. Know that your vision is not just a fantasy, it's your dream with a plan attached.

Day Fourteen
Do the Right Thing

"Real integrity is doing the right thing, knowing that nobody's going to know
whether you did it or not."
Oprah Winfrey

Are you an honest person? I know you are. But are you honest with yourself? Will you do what's right for you to succeed? Will you stick to your plan? That's the integral thing to do, if you want to have a different life. If you want to have the life you imagine.

I see people want success in business, health and relationships. But they aren't doing what it takes to make those dreams a reality. Is honesty wanting or expecting something we won't work for? Is it honest for me to post my goals for a happy, balanced, well-rounded life, when I'm not doing anything to achieve those goals?

We've been on the 30-day journey for a couple of weeks now. Truthfully, are you sticking to your plan? Are you really working to make this year better than the last? Or did you waste your money buying this book? I'm asking, because I want you to be honest. Ask yourself right now, "Am I doing the right thing?"

Ignorance is no longer an excuse. Lack of education and inspiration is no longer a reason for you not reaching your full potential. Imagine the life you want to live. See how you will be better and how your family and friends will see that change. You have a plan to succeed. Now work that plan.

Day Fifteen
Visualize to Actualize

"See things as you would have them be instead of as they are."
Robert Collier

Imagination is vital to your success. It's not just for artists or children. It's for you and me, as well. A vivid imagination can help us see ourselves living the life we want to live.

Another word for imagination is visualization. It means imagining a scene, a person or an object with intense clarity. Intense clarity. That means you can see, smell and feel your new life!

Visualization works. I use it all the time. I imagined I would earn $100,000 in a 12-month period in Pre-Paid Legal and wear the 6-figure ring. I visualized myself giving my acceptance speech on stage. I memorized my speech two years before I actually gave it! Almost every day, I saw myself standing on stage. I saw my hair, my dress, I even heard myself dedicating the ring to my father. I didn't just see it. I lived it, over and over again. I got the 6-figure ring two years after I started visualizing it.

What do you really want? Are you visualizing yourself with it? Here are some steps to using this technique for your success:

1. Find a quiet, private place. Visualize in bed, in front of the bathroom mirror, the closet. It doesn't matter. I believe in visualizing in private. You don't want anyone or anything messing up your success scenes.

2.   Relax. Breathe. Get loose. Let go of the tension of the present so you can see the success of the future.

3.   Engage your senses. First, decide what you want. Then picture the idea or object exactly how you want it to be. Then place yourself in that scene. See yourself in the clothes you're wearing. Hear the applause. Feel the wind in your hair. I don't know what you want; but vividly imagine getting it.

4.   Believe. You must have faith that you can have it. This isn't fantasizing you're doing. This is foreshadowing. You're just seeing it before it actually happens. You can't have any doubt your dreams will come true.

5.   Visualize your success every day. Your subconscious has to be reminded regularly of what's to come. No matter what's going on in your life, take time to see your success that's on the way. The more you see it, the more you'll believe it.

I have visualized myself with so many things that have come true! I have seen myself in outfits I have worn, my first home, my dream car and my wedding day. I've gotten so good at visualizing; I have to stop myself sometimes! Because if I can see it, I can achieve it! And you can too!

Day Sixteen
It's All or Nothing

"To get what you want, you must be prepared not to have it at all."

There's a quote from the movie, *The Untouchables*, where Malone says to Elliott Ness, "If you open the can on these worms you must be prepared to go all the way." You've opened this can of worms, now, you have to go all the way.

Once the mind expands, it can never go back to its original dimension. You can't go back now, you know too much. You've improved too much. You've gotten a taste of your new life; you can't possible go back to your previous, ordinary existence.

I went on a zip line excursion with some friends in Puerto Vallarta, Mexico. The scenery was beautiful, while at times a little unnerving. We were hundreds of feet in the air. We had to hike for miles to get to the zip lines, crossing some of the most beautiful landscape I'd ever seen. The tour guide told us that many people didn't want to hike, (the hard part), to get to the zip lines, (the fun part). He said he watched many people hike for miles, work extremely hard and miss out on the zip line, the best part: because they were tired or afraid, they would give up. They had to hike back to the starting point. More hard work. He said, "They spent more time giving up and turning around, than if they kept hiking to their destination. The zip line was what they were working for; they missed that by giving up."

That resonated with me. Many of us are like that. We'll spend more time complaining and quitting, than pressing on to reach our goals. You've come too far on this 30 day journey…it's harder to give up than it is to succeed. Press on. Beautiful scenery is just ahead.

Day Seventeen
Finish What You've Started

"The more you start over, the longer it takes to achieve your success. Life is too short for multiple beginnings."

I feel we've all been put on this earth to accomplish something significant. We have a set amount of time to get it done. When we start something and quit, start something and quit, start something and quit again, we're spinning our wheels. We're getting nowhere. The people whose lives will be changed by our gift are being cheated.

Whether you believe it or not, you have something the world needs. Sticking to your plan to succeed doesn't just help you; it helps others you've never met, whose names you don't even know.

We can't accomplish what God has for us to do in our lifetime. That's why He gives us children. They will continue our work after we are gone. That's powerful! That means when we are successful our children are better equipped to continue the work God has for us, for our families. My Dad used to say, "My job is to raise you to be good citizens that can make a contribution to impact the world." That was rather profound for a man that worked in a manufacturing plant canning beer. It was profound and right on target. Because that's what he did. Even though he's not alive to see it, I am a good citizen. I am making contributions to society; and I'm just getting started on impacting the world.

You need to have a big vision like my father. Whether you have children or not, you have family, friends, co-workers or employees who can help take your gift to the world. But it starts with you. It starts today.

Don't quit. There are too many people counting on you to finish this time, not start all over again.

Day Eighteen
Enough is Enough

"How can you be too weak to make the break, but strong enough to keep bearing the pain?"

This quote reminds me of a story about a dog on a nail. A man walked to work every day. He passed barking dogs every day. But there was one dog he would pass that never barked. She would only moan, groan and whimper. He passed these dogs every day for a week. All the dogs would bark; but that one dog would only whimper. One day, the man got fed up. He decided to find out why this dog only moaned and never barked. When he came to where the whimpering dog lived, he asked the owner, "Why does your dog moan and whimper, while the other dogs bark?" The owner said, "Because she's sitting on a nail." The man said, "What? That's got to hurt! Why doesn't she get off?" The owner said, "I guess it doesn't hurt her enough yet."

Are you like the whimpering dog? Are you man or woman enough to take the pain; but not man or woman enough to end it? Do you let everyone know how bad your situation is, but won't do anything about it? Today that ends! You will not go another day voicing your woes to the world. You will let the world see you as an overcomer.

You have the plan, now work it. Stop complaining and start doing. Get off that nail! God meant your life to be more comfortable than that!

Tiffaney Beverly Malott

(lined blank page)

Day Nineteen
Don't Hide, Face Yourself!

"The one person you can't run from is yourself."

We can run from a lot of things...people, exercise, responsibilities. But we can't run from the truth. And the truth is in each of us. When you look in the mirror, the person looking back at you knows if you've been sticking to your plan. That person knows if you're taking the steps to a greater life. That person also knows if you're not.

We all slip sometimes. Sometimes we just fall down. We just have to get up again. Proverbs 24:16, (Bible in Basic English translation), says, "For an upright man, after falling seven times, will get up again..." Have you gotten off course? Have you let distractions take you off your path to success? It's okay. Just ask yourself: What was it? Why did it I let it happen? How can I keep from letting it happen again? Stand back up, brush yourself off and start walking down your path to victory.

The one person you'll always have to live with is you. Will you be able to live with yourself if you quit? Will you be able to live with yourself if you give up? Do you have the courage to face yourself? Remember, "Courage doesn't always roar. Sometimes, it's the quiet voice at the end of the day saying, 'I will try again tomorrow.'" Mary Ann Radmacher.

Tiffaney Beverly Malott

Day Twenty
D.I.Y. – Do it Yourself!

"God gave you food, but He didn't cook it. He gave you fruit, but He didn't pick it. He gave you the cow, but He didn't kill it. Some things you've got to do yourself."

In today's HGTV/Food Network world, many of us "know" how to build a deck, redesign a house and bake a soufflé. We vicariously experience success through the hard work of others. I think God gave us this life to experience for ourselves. We're supposed to learn from, not live through, the experiences of someone else.

Our life is supposed to be DO IT YOURSELF. Stop hoping and waiting; and start learning and doing. Good things happen to those who ACT! We can't be healthy sitting on the couch with a remote in our hands watching people work out. We can't work from home if we don't work the opportunity we have in front of us. We can't change the world if we don't change ourselves.

When it comes to D.I.Y., there are some things we must consider.

1. Skills. You must be realistic about your skills. Don't try to take on work that you won't be able to finish. You can partner with someone with more skills than you. That way you can still get the job done right, even though you're not a pro at it yet.

2. Tools. Be aware that you'll need tools. Certain jobs require certain tools. The great thing about D.I.Y. in life is that the tools are all around:

bookstores, libraries, websites and people. You just have to look for them. When the student is ready, the teacher will appear.

3. Time. Don't forget to take time into consideration. Even spare time has a value. Apply the slight edge principle. A few simple disciplines practiced over time changes everything! Remember, in life, a little bit of time each day can add more years and more fulfillment to your existence.

After taking these three things into consideration, don't forget there is another option. You can do some of the work yourself and save the more complicated tasks for the pros. In other words, remember to cast God in you D.I.Y. life production. Some things He meant for you to do. The other things He's already taken care of for you.

This is your life. You want to make it great? You've got to Do It Yourself.

_____

_____

_____

_____

_____

_____

_____

_____

_____

_____

_____

_____

_____

Day Twenty-One
Feed Your Mind with Empowering Information

"Pour your purse into your mind and your mind will pour back into your purse."

John Malott's take on Ben Franklin's actual quote

GIGO. Garbage In. Garbage Out. I learned this acronym in middle school. It means if you put bad programming into a computer, bad programming will come out of the computer. Your mind is the world's most advanced computer. What programming are you putting in it? Is it hours of pop and hip-hop songs? Is it racy novels? Or is it every episode of Dancing with the Stars, American Idol, Grey's Anatomy or Desperate Housewives?

Remember, what you put in is what you get out! I'm not saying these songs, books or TV shows are bad. Okay. Change that. That is what I'm saying. The majority of pop culture isn't helping us win in life. It's a shame to me when the conversation of a thirty-something woman is all about trashy novels, the latest episode of reality television and music videos. She can't really be positive, because nothing positive is going in her. A weekly dose of religion is just not enough. What your spouse, significant other, friends or pastor is reading is not enough either. What are you pouring into your mind? You don't become successful through osmosis.

You need positive, motivational, educational, inspirational information daily! You can read books, listen to audio CD's, plug into conference calls or go

43

to events. People may not like this stuff; but I love it. I've found that people who don't like these things are usually living the life we don't want to live.

I used to be a very negative person. For me, the glass was half empty and it had a hole in the bottom. I was a pessimist and proud of it. I thought I was just being real. I was just being my environment. I listened to music with not-so-positive lyrics. I read books that didn't have good messages. I watched shows that didn't make me a better person. Combine those factors with my negative friends and co-workers, I was a walking abyss of negativity. I wasn't very happy and didn't know why. Then I was introduced to Pre-Paid Legal and personal development. Now, I'm happy, upbeat and a source of positivity for others.

What's on your life's programming schedule? Remember GIGO. Garbage In. Garbage Out. I think it's time to take out the trash.

Day Twenty-Two
Dress for Success

"Clothes make the man. Naked people have little or no influence in society."

Mark Twain

Naked or inappropriately dressed people have little or no influence in society. Let's be real. How you dress does matter. Think about the most attractive people you know. Do you think they'd be as attractive with no clothes on? Okay. You're right. Some of them would. But you and I both know their style has a lot to do with it. Hello...Snap out of it! Stop thinking about them with no clothes on!

Dressing for success doesn't mean looking like some model in a magazine. It means kickin' butt, taking names and looking absolutely fierce while doing it. I read that style is the distinctive way you speak, act and dress. Find your style. Not someone else's. It's a shame to see people not dressing their age. They are over thirty and look they raided their 15-year olds closet. You can be professional, sexy and age appropriate.

Look your best at all times, at work and at play. If you look good, you'll do even better. That doesn't mean you have to go out and buy lots of clothes. I bet you can look great with what's in your closet right now.

Your attitude is also part of your success wardrobe. It is your ambassador to the world. Your smile, your tone and how you treat people is part of getting dressed every day. You could have on designer apparel from head to toe. If you are a b____, well you know. Your clothes won't matter at all.

45

So, no matter what your money, business or family situation looks like...put on your success wardrobe and go change your world. It's true: if you look good, you'll feel good; and if you feel good you can do incredible things!

Day Twenty-Three
Let Your Light Shine!

"Never dull your shine for someone else."

Tyra Banks

My husband said, "If you want people to love you...fail." Just be mediocre and status quo. You'll stay popular, but will you be happy and fulfilled? Playing yourself down, helps no one. I know it can be hard. Some of us are nurturers. We want to help everybody. We want everyone to be a winner. But, can I bring you into the real world? Do I have your permission to break this thing down? It's survival of the fittest, sweetie; which can be simply rewritten as "survival of those that are better equipped for surviving." So everyone won't make it, because everyone won't work to better equip themselves. In other words, everyone won't make it with you. Some people will be left behind. Not because you don't care; because they don't want to come.

I heard a friend say, "Some people won't participate in their own rescue." That doesn't mean you throw your life preserver away and drown with them! SUCCEED! They will still be there. You help no one by not being your best. The greatest thing you can do for your naysayers, aka friends and family members, is to not be afraid to be the best you can be. By doing that, you'll give them the courage to be more themselves. Billy Graham said, "When a brave man takes a stand, the spines of others stiffen." Are you brave enough to stand for your success, your financial independence, your gift to the world?

Marianne Williamson said, "You playing small doesn't serve the world…As we are liberated from our own fear, our presence automatically liberates others." Free yourself, free the world.

_____

_____

_____

_____

_____

_____

_____

_____

_____

_____

_____

_____

_____

_____

_____

_____

_____

_____

_____

_____

_____

_____

Day Twenty-Four
Shake it Off!

"Gotta do what's best for me; Baby that means I gotta shake you off."

"Shake It Off", Mariah Carey

I don't know who Mariah was talking too; but she hit the nail on the head. We've got to learn to 'shake it off'. I have a tendency to hold on to things, especially things that have hurt me. The longer I hold onto it, the more it festers inside me. It poisons my spirit and saps my joy.

Hopefully, you don't know what I'm talking about. If you do, shake it off. Pop it off your collar. Flick it off your shoulder. Shake your hips. Do all those dances the kids do that means they're not going to worry or be affected by anything. I'm not just talking about shaking off relationship drama. Shake off all your drama! Shake off your crazy family, trifling friends, your bad ass kids, your hectic job, your crazy boss, your slow-growing business and any other drama life throws your way. Don't let it get to you!

We've got to stop taking everything so personally! How do we do that when someone was rude to me? Or he just doesn't love me anymore? When they chose someone else for the promotion instead of me? They did these things to me. That's all personal, right?

The operative word in these scenarios is ME. When someone else is doing or saying something to you, it's about them, not you! Say, "It's about THEM, not about ME!" If you hear yourself say, "I can't believe they did or said that to ME," stop and realize you used the word ME about someone else's behavior.

49

Don't make yourself the important part of the interaction. It's about them and how they are acting. It's not about you.

Easier said than done, right? Here's another way to shake it off and not take things so personally. Work on healing your wounds. As we heal, we can better see other people's wounds that make them act in all sorts of ways. Often we can't see someone else's pain because our wounds are too tender. They hit a nerve with us, we react and now we think it's about us. Start working on healing yourself. What are some things you need healing on today?

The two ways to shake it off and not take things personally is: 1. Remember it's not about you. 2. Heal yourself. You can stay the victim or you can become the victor. It's your choice.

_____

_____

_____

_____

_____

_____

_____

_____

_____

_____

_____

_____

Day Twenty-Five
Know Your Value

"Who you are is more important than what you have. So, what you become is more significant than what you acquire."

Bishop Noel Jones

I read in *Why We Want You to be Rich* by Donald Trump and Robert Kiyosaki, "Americans always know the price; they very rarely know the value." When writing this, I wondered, "Do I know the difference?" So I did a little research and this is what I found.

- Cost-is the amount you spend to produce your product or service
- Price-is your financial reward for providing your product or service
- Value-is what your customer believes the product or service is worth

Let's look at me as an example: The cost for me to be where I am today has been minimal. I invested $249 in a home-based business opportunity that has changed my life. I have invested money along the way. Over the past eight years, I would guess that it's been less than $50,000. I invested time as well. Was it a lot? I don't think I had to invest any new time. I just redirected the time I was spending somewhere else to changing the rest of my life. So I turned off the TV, the radio, my negative friends and family. I turned on positive books and audio programs. That was the cost. Was it worth it? Well, you tell me.

The price, my financial reward for paying the above costs are as follows: I achieved a 6-figure annual income from home in only three years of paying the costs. I earn a multiple 6-figure income from home today. I earn more money in a month than I used to earn in a year. I am a 35-year old millionaire. I work from home. I vacation almost every month. I have the time to take part in different volunteer opportunities in my area. I live the life I always dreamed. Looking good so far...

The value is priceless. No, really. I can't put a price tag on the value of my life today. Because I get a chance to live this way, I get a chance to help more people. I believe my value to the world will outweigh my price and my cost combined. It's what I will give, not what I get, that will determine my true value to others.

I understand my value and my increasing value today. But it wasn't always like that. I used to equate my value to what assets I had acquired. I thought the more money I made, the more I was worth. I thought that made me more important in the eyes of others. I was so wrong! I've learned that more assets don't determine my value. My contribution to the world does. The people that led the greatest movements of all time were probably not wearing Gucci or Prada and driving a BMW. They realized their impact on the world had nothing to do with their bank account. You can start changing the world from where you are right now. What you have doesn't matter. What you do with it does. You're valuable right now. Make sure you know your value so you can let the world know.

Day Twenty-Six
Discover Your Talent

"Your talent is God's gift to you. What you do with it is your gift back to God."

Leo Buscaglia

Have you found your talent? Have you discovered your gift to the world? Eight years ago, I would've laughed out loud if someone had asked me that. I would have probably said, "I do my job well, so I guess I've found my talent. I make damn good jelly."

But that wasn't my talent. That was part of the process to discovering my talent. I didn't find joy in making jelly. I found joy in communicating with people. I found joy in helping them become better so they could perform better. That was my talent, not making jelly.

Can you relate? You're good at what you do, so you think that's got to be your talent. It doesn't bring you true joy or fulfillment; but because you can do it in your sleep, you stick with it. That's not your talent. That's your vocation, a job you're suited or qualified for. That's not your avocation, which is something you do that makes you happy. You've probably heard, "work part-time on your fortune, while you work full-time on your job." I have found that most people amass huge fortunes working their avocations/what they love. People with no fortunes spend all their time on their vocation/job.

A synonym of talent is endowment. I like that term, so I'll go further. An endowment is a gift accepted with donor stipulations. God gave you a gift, but there are stipulations. A stipulation is a course of action mutually agreed upon.

God has given you the gift, now you must take action. As you improve in all areas of your life, doors will open for you that will allow you to work your talent and give your gift to the world.

The Pre-Paid Legal opportunity, along with personal development, helped me grow from the inside out. It was the refining process that allowed me to discover my talent and my true joy. Let our 30-day journey together, be part of your process to discovering and using your talents.

_____

_____

_____

_____

_____

_____

_____

_____

_____

_____

_____

_____

_____

_____

_____

_____

_____

_____

Day Twenty-Seven
It Had to Come to This

"Sometimes you have to almost lose your mind before you change your mind."

Have you ever asked yourself, "How did this happen?" or "How did I get here?" I don't know how you got where you are, but I do know two things: 1. It didn't happen overnight. 2. You don't have to stay there.

God may have let you get to this point so you can finally hear Him! Now that He's gotten your attention: LISTEN! Don't take your hardships or difficult situations personally. Be excited about the challenges, because they are just opportunities for you to grow. You're being prepared for your next level.

Some bumblebees were taken along on a space mission for a study on the effects of weightlessness. Similar to humans in space, the bees floated around with such great ease, they didn't even have to use their wings. It looked as though they were thriving in the weightless environment without work, struggle or adversity. But after three days, all the bees died. The experiment was summed up with these words: "They enjoyed the ride, but they didn't survive."

How a bee flies is a mystery to scientists. A bee shouldn't be able to fly. Its body is too big and its wings are too short. But they fly any way; except in space. The bees died when they didn't have to work to live. They died when they didn't have any resistance. You're just like those bees with their too-big bodies and short wings. People are wondering how you're making it. How are you raising those kids on your own? How are you thriving in your business while dealing with an unsupportive spouse? How are you sending your kids to the best school while working a job and running a business? People are marveling at you the way scientists marvel at the bees. They are wondering how you're making it on those short wings? You're making it because you are using your resistance to propel you upward. We weren't meant to go through life with no resistance. The challenges, hardships and difficulties are only making you stronger so you can soar higher.

_____

_____

_____

_____

_____

_____

_____

_____

_____

_____

_____

_____

_____

_____

_____

_____

Day Twenty-Eight
Pay Yourself First

"Who you work for is waiting for you at home."

Our employers may think we go to work every day for the company's mission statement or serving the customers. But the real reason we go to work is for us; for the sake of ourselves and our families. We go to work for the well-being of those we love. Everything else is secondary.

Or do we? Most of us haven't been raised to put ourselves first. We are raised to be nice, to share and to help others. That's what we do. We nicely pay our share of our check to help others live betters lives than we do. I know that stung a little bit; but it's true.

We have to start paying ourselves first. The wealthy do this with no reservation. I read on a website that if this is all you do, pay yourself first, you can be rich. If you do what most Americans don't, you can have what most Americans won't. Stop paying the credit card company, the landlord, the telephone company and the government first. Pay you first.

People devise budgets to figure out how to pay everyone else by the end of each month; and give themselves the leftovers. This is financially backwards! If you are doing this, stop right now. Put money aside for yourself at the beginning of every month or every pay period. Make this a habit. If you don't, you'll make more, spend more and still be broke.

There is more you need to learn. How much should you pay yourself, where you should put your money, etc. I suggest reading financial books and websites. One book I suggest is *Smart Women Finish Rich*, *Smart Couples Finish Rich* or *Automatic Millionaire* by David Bach. Also read *The Richest Man in Babylon* by George S. Clayson. These are great books, with a lot of priceless information. These aren't the only books out there on this topic; but they helped me immensely.

I just want you to get this philosophy down. Pay yourself first! Here's a scenario: You're in a desert for many days and you have no food or water. You come across an oasis full of water and delicious food. Would you put the water in bottles and put the food in to-go boxes and send them to other people you owe food and water? Or would you get your fill first? This illustration may have been a little too simple. Maybe I'm being just a bit obvious with my message here. But you get the picture. Take care of you first. The landlord, the tax man and the telephone customer service rep will still be there.

Day Twenty-Nine
I'm Careful about What I Say

"The tongue is like a sharp knife…Kills without drawing blood."

Buddha

There is an old proverb with a lot of wisdom. It says, "The tongue has the power of life and death…" We all know this to be true. How many of us have been on the wrong side of a sharp tongue? Some of us are affected to this day by someone else's evil tongue. We must be careful what we say to everyone we come in contact with. It's so easy to be flippant and irresponsible with our words. I know this all too well. I learned the importance of a kind tongue too late in my life. My tongue, as a weapon, has left a lot of carnage. I've hurt people and in some cases, didn't even realize it; or didn't care to. Have you ever done that? Hurt someone with your words out of anger, malice or jest? It doesn't just hurt them, it hurts us too. We must learn to be responsible with our words. Think before we speak. Take a deep breath or walk away. Respond, don't react. Stop thinking we need to give someone a piece of our mind.

I also want you to be more careful about what you say to yourself. Some of us commit suicide daily with our tongues. We wonder why things aren't better in our lives. It's because we speak negative things to ourselves about ourselves.

Stop saying you're ugly, poor and destined to fail. You can be honest about your situation; but still positive. So what, you're overweight. Just say, "I need to drop some weight. But damn I'm fine while I'm losing it!" Your checking account may be a mess. Say to yourself, "This check may have

59

bounced, but only I can make insufficient funds look this good!" Maybe you missed your goals for your business again! Repeat this quote by George Bernard Shaw, "a life spent making mistakes is not only more honorable but more useful than a life spent doing nothing." Think to yourself, "My mistakes are honorable and useful!"

The words you use on yourself create things in you, positive things or negative things. What you speak to yourself is your choice. Choose to use your tongue as a positive force for your life and the lives of those you love.

_____

_____

_____

_____

_____

_____

_____

_____

_____

_____

_____

_____

_____

_____

_____

_____

_____

Day Thirty
Enjoy the Journey

"Life is the journey and the journey is life."

We must be at peace with where we are right now. We may have some areas we need to improve in; but we need to look at our situation and be thankful for what we are and where we are. Sometimes we forget that there will always be some distance between where we are and where we want to be. So we must learn to enjoy the journey between these two points. Where you are now is just a step to where you want to go. When you reach the next level, it will be just a step to another level and so on. Each level is the first step of another adventure and off you grow again.

The best way to live is to find joy in the present. As Abraham-Hicks teaches, "if you're not feeling good, if you're not having fun, if you're not enjoying the journey, you're really missing the point of being here."

This concludes our thirty days together. But it's just the beginning of your journey. Your life will be everything you want because you've seen it, spoken it and worked it. Please stick with it. Don't let anyone take you off your course. Success, in all areas of your life, is yours.

Stay humble, stay disciplined, stay prayerful, but most of all, stay you.

Conclusion

What do we do now? We start all over on the next thirty days of your life. You don't need this book any more to become a better you. But I do hope this book helped you realize how easy it is to start on your personal, success journey.

The next step is to evaluate your progress over the past thirty days. How did you do? Do you see any change? It doesn't matter how small the change is, just as long as it's in the right direction. Now we need to set new goals for the next thirty days. Your next set of goals can be a continuation of the first set; or they can be the next step for you. Don't be afraid to stretch yourself. Remember to write your goals; make them specific, make them visible and make them a reality.

Congratulations on completing these thirty days! Most people give up, get distracted or make excuses why they can't succeed. You didn't do any of these things. There is only one more thing you must do. You must find another Mordecai. My task is finished; but there are others waiting to help you on your journey. Find another book with a positive message; put an audio program in your car. Immerse yourself in the teachings. They will take you to another level.

If this information was helpful, let me know. Give me a call: 877-270-1197.Leave me a message. Or you can visit my website: www.tlotti.com. Please leave me a comment. Visit regularly, because I have a blog and trainings that can help you on your continued journey.

I am grateful to you for allowing me, in my own way, to touch your life. Now, in your own way, please go touch the lives of others.

Tiffaney Beverly Malott

Notes

Tiffaney Beverly Malott